CONTROLLING

HIGH BLOOD PRESSURE

Natural Remedies & Lifestyle Changes

By

Joseph Ihekwoaba

TABLE OF CONTENTS

INTRODUCTION

In today's fast-paced society, when stress and unhealthy habits seem to saturate our everyday lives, high blood pressure appears as a silent but formidable health opponent.

Millions of individuals throughout the world struggle with high blood pressure, which puts their cardiovascular health in danger. The good news is that by using natural treatments and making healthy lifestyle changes, we have the amazing potential to regulate this ailment.

We can start a transformational path toward a better, more satisfying life by realizing the potential that already exists inside us. When the blood's strain on our artery walls continuously exceeds what is normal, high blood pressure develops.

If untreated, it can lead to major side effects including stroke, heart attack, and renal problems. While pharmaceuticals can be an important part of managing hypertension, a natural approach that emphasizes utilizing the body's innate healing capacities offers a compelling alternative.

In this age of empowerment and personal development, it is critical to recognize that we possess the key to our overall well-being. While there is no doubt that medical interventions have their place, natural remedies, and lifestyle changes give us the chance to reclaim control over our health.

We set out on a fantastic journey to a healthy, more vibrant existence by fueling our bodies with the blessings of nature, establishing regular exercise routines, controlling stress, and quitting unhealthy behaviors.

We shall explore the interesting world of natural treatments and lifestyle modifications that can help us defeat high blood pressure in the pages that follow.

We will arm ourselves with the knowledge and tools necessary to take charge of our health destiny through the investigation of evidence-based tactics and useful advice.

Let's collectively discover our inner strength and set out on a revolutionary journey to reach our highest level of wellness, when high blood pressure becomes a thing of the past and vitality becomes our everyday reality.

CHAPTER 1

Definition of High Blood Pressure

High blood pressure, which is also referred to as hypertension, is a prevalent health issue in which the blood is constantly pushing against the artery walls.

If left untreated, this can put an excessive amount of stress on the heart and blood vessels, which could result in serious health issues.

About one in three adults in the United States has high blood pressure, making it a significant public health issue. High blood pressure is common, but many people with it have no symptoms, which is why it's often called the "silent killer."

High Blood Pressure Symptoms

Regular blood pressure checks are crucial because, as was already mentioned, high blood pressure frequently has no apparent symptoms. But occasionally, those who have high blood pressure may exhibit signs like:

- Headaches

- Breathing difficulty

- Nosebleeds

- Fatigue

- Chest discomfort

These signs and symptoms are not unique to high blood pressure and can be brought on by other illnesses. For a correct diagnosis, it is crucial to speak with a healthcare professional.

Causes of High Blood Pressure

The precise reason for high blood pressure is typically unknown. However, many factors may play a role in the condition's emergence. These consist of:

1. Age: As arteries become stiffer and more constricted with time, blood pressure tends to rise with age.

2. Genetics: The likelihood of developing high blood pressure is increased if there is a family history of the condition.

3. Lifestyle factors: Unhealthy practices like a diet high in salt and saturated fats, inactivity, and excessive alcohol consumption can cause high blood pressure.

4. Obesity: Being obese can put additional stress on the heart and blood vessels, which can raise blood pressure.

5. Medical conditions: Diabetes, kidney disease, and sleep apnea are some conditions that can raise the risk of developing high blood pressure.

High Blood Pressure Complications

Untreated high blood pressure can result in several serious health issues, such as:

1. Heart disease: High blood pressure makes the heart work harder than it needs to, which increases the likelihood of heart disease.

2. Stroke: High blood pressure can result in brain blood vessels bursting or blocking, which can result in a stroke.

3. Kidney disease: Over time, kidney damage brought on by high blood pressure can develop.

4. Loss of vision: Blood vessels in the eyes can become damaged by high blood pressure, which impairs vision.

5. Erectile dysfunction: In men, erectile dysfunction can be brought on by high blood pressure.

High Blood Pressure Treatment

The following are examples of lifestyle modifications that can lower blood pressure:

1. Eating a balanced diet low in saturated fats and salt

2. Physical activity regularly

3. Being healthy in terms of weight

4. Restricting alcohol intake

5. Giving up smoking

Along with modifying one's lifestyle, many medications, including the ones listed below, can be used to treat high blood pressure:

1. Diuretics: By assisting the body in flushing out extra water and sodium, these drugs help to lower blood pressure and reduce blood volume.

2. ACE inhibitors: These drugs prevent the synthesis of the hormone angiotensin II, which can constrict blood vessels and raise blood pressure.

3. Calcium channel blockers: These drugs ease blood vessel tension, facilitating easier blood flow and lowering blood pressure.

4. Beta-blockers: These drugs counteract the effects of adrenaline, which lowers blood pressure and heart rate.

The ideal treatment strategy for controlling high blood pressure should be determined in collaboration with a healthcare professional.

To monitor blood pressure and make sure that treatment is working, regular blood pressure checks are also necessary.

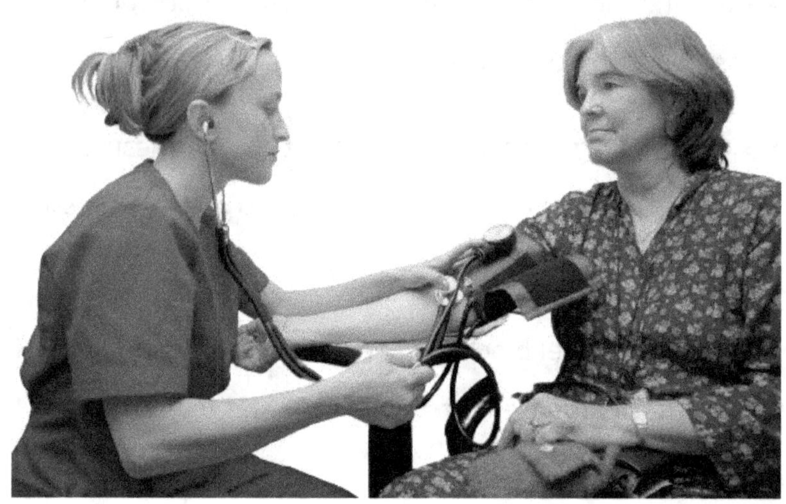

CHAPTER 2

Diagnosis of High Blood Pressure

For early detection and treatment of hypertension, it is crucial to go for a routine blood pressure check. According to the Center for Disease Control and Prevention (CDC), high blood pressure kills about 1,000 Americans per day.

It is estimated that one-third of persons in the US have hypertension, yet many are unaware of it because they show no symptoms.

Individuals who are at risk of having high blood pressure can be identified through blood pressure screenings, enabling them to take precautions to lower their risk.

Regular blood pressure checks are necessary for people who have already received a diagnosis of high blood pressure in order to monitor the level of their blood pressure and make sure their treatment is working.

How To Check Your Blood Pressure

A sphygmomanometer, which is made up of an inflatable cuff, a pressure gauge, and a stethoscope, is used to measure blood pressure. Systolic and diastolic readings are the two different kinds of blood pressure measurements.

Systolic blood pressure gauges the force exerted by the heart as it pumps blood through the arteries. Diastolic blood pressure gauges how much pressure is present in the arteries between heartbeats.

Your upper arm is wrapped in a cuff that is inflated until the artery contracts in order to take your blood pressure. After hearing the sound of blood flowing through the artery with a stethoscope, the pressure is then progressively relaxed.

The location where the sound stops and restarts represents the systolic blood pressure, while the location where the sound starts and stops represents the diastolic blood pressure.

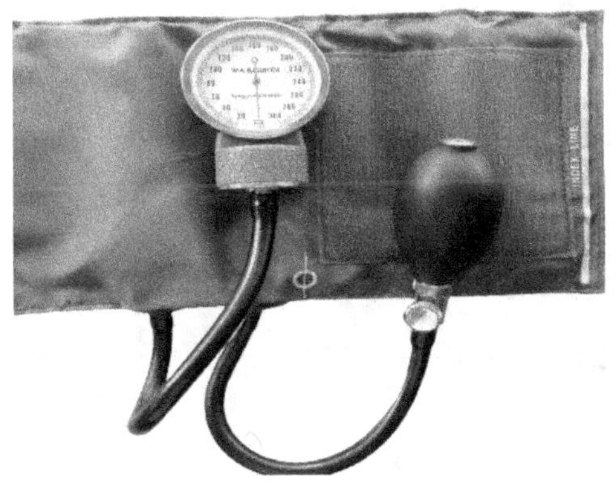

Blood Pressure Reading Classifications

There are four categories for blood pressure readings: normal, elevated, stage 1 hypertension, and stage 2 hypertension.

Normal blood pressure is when the systolic reading is below 120mm Hg, and the diastolic reading is below 80mm Hg.

Elevated blood pressure is when the systolic value is between 120 and 129mm Hg and a diastolic value that is less than 80mm Hg.

Stage 1 hypertension is a systolic value that is between 130-139 mm Hg or a diastolic value that is between 80-89 mm Hg.

Stage 2 hypertension is a systolic value of 140 mm Hg or higher or a diastolic value of 90 mm Hg or higher.

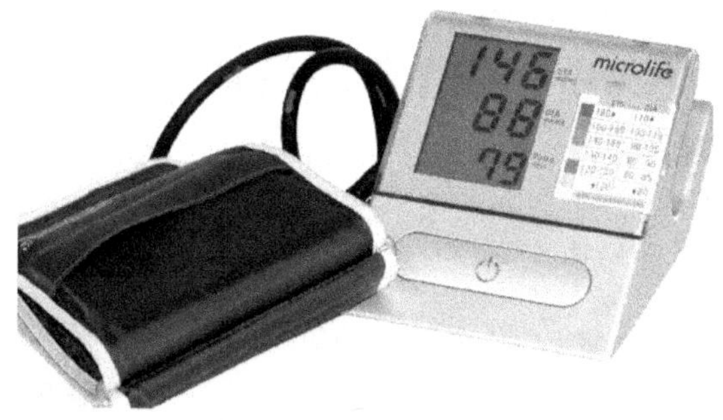

The Right Time to Seek Medical Help

If your blood pressure level is high, it's imperative to seek medical assistance immediately.

Although minor cases of high blood pressure may not require immediate treatment, it is still vital to check your readings frequently and implement lifestyle changes to lower your blood pressure.

CHAPTER 3

Medical Management of Hypertension

Even though healthy eating habits and regular exercise can lower blood pressure, some people may also need to take medication.

High Blood Pressure Medications

Many different drug classes are frequently used to treat high blood pressure. These consist of:

1. Diuretics: Diuretics, often known as water pills, are drugs that aid in the removal of excess water and salt from the human body. As a result, the blood arteries hold less fluid, which can assist in lowering blood pressure. Diuretics are classified as thiazide, loop, or potassium-sparing.

2.ACE inhibitors: By preventing the generation of the hormone angiotensin II, ACE inhibitors, also known as angiotensin-converting enzyme inhibitors, help to relax blood vessels and reduce blood pressure.

3. Angiotensin receptor blockers (ARBs): ARBs are drugs that inhibit the activity of angiotensin II, thereby helping to relax blood vessels and reduce blood pressure.

4. Calcium channel blockers: By limiting the quantity of calcium that goes into the cells of the blood vessels and heart, calcium channel blockers work to calm the blood vessels.

5. Beta-blockers: Beta-blockers are drugs that help to control blood pressure by lowering the heart rate and the volume of blood the heart pumps.

6. Alpha-blockers: Alpha-blockers are drugs that aid in blood vessel muscle relaxation, which can lower blood pressure.

Potential Negative Effects Of Medications

Despite their potential for managing high blood pressure, medicines can have negative side effects. Some of the most prevalent negative effects of blood pressure medicines are:

1. Diuretics: Diuretics may result in electrolyte imbalances, low blood potassium levels, and dehydration.

2.ACE inhibitors: ACE inhibitors may result in a rash, a dry cough, and dizziness.

3.ARBs: ARBs have been linked to headaches, diarrhea, and vertigo.

4. Calcium channel blockers: These medications can make you feel lightheaded, give you headaches, and make your ankles and feet swell.

5. Beta-blockers: Beta-blockers have been linked to impotence, drowsiness, and weariness.

6. Alpha-blockers: These medications have the potential to make you weak and dizzy.

Alternative Therapies

Other than traditional medical methods, there are a variety of alternative therapies that can lower blood pressure. They include:

1. Lifestyle changes can help lower blood pressure. These include eating a nutritious diet, exercising regularly, keeping a healthy weight, and decreasing stress.

2. Supplements: Some dietary supplements, including coenzyme Q10, omega-3 fatty acids, and garlic, may help decrease blood pressure.

3. Meditation: By reducing stress, meditation and other relaxation methods may help to reduce blood pressure.

4. Biofeedback: Biofeedback is a practice that involves employing electronic instruments to help control biological functions such as blood pressure. People may be capable to lower their blood pressure by comprehending how to control these functions.

5. Yoga: By increasing relaxation and lowering stress levels, practicing yoga helps lower blood pressure.

It is crucial to remember that even while these complementary therapies may be beneficial for some people, they shouldn't be taken in place of medication without first consulting a healthcare professional.

CHAPTER 4

Blood Pressure Lowering Diet

Making dietary modifications can be a useful strategy for controlling blood pressure.

The significance of a healthy diet for controlling blood pressure

For maintaining ideal blood pressure levels, a nutritious diet is crucial. The following dietary recommendations are provided by the American Heart Association for managing blood pressure:

1. Eat a variety of vegetables, fruits, whole grains, and low-fat dairy products.

2. Limit consumption of saturated and trans fats, salt, cholesterol, and added sugars

3. Choose lean protein sources such as fish, poultry, beans, and nuts

4. Limit consumption of red meat and processed meats

5. Choose healthy fats such as olive oil, nuts, and avocados

6. Limit alcohol consumption

High Blood Pressure DASH Diet

The DASH (Dietary Approaches to Stop Hypertension) diet is one of the best for lowering blood pressure. While limiting trans and saturated fats, cholesterol, salt, and added sugars, this diet emphasizes whole foods like lean protein, vegetables, whole grains, fruits, and low-fat dairy products.

In as little as two weeks, the DASH diet can considerably lower blood pressure readings, according to research that was published in the New England Journal of Medicine.

The DASH diet was also proven to lower blood pressure levels more effectively than a low-sodium diet, according to the study.

High Blood Pressure Foods To Avoid

It's crucial to avoid some foods that can raise blood pressure levels in addition to maintaining a balanced diet. These consist of:

1. Salt: Consuming too much sodium might cause fluid retention and raised blood pressure. For persons with hypertension or at risk for hypertension, the recommended daily sodium consumption is 1,500 milligrams, which is lower than the recommended daily sodium intake of 2,300 mg.

2. Processed meals: Processed foods, like canned soups, frozen dinners, and packaged snacks, frequently include a lot of added sugar and sodium.

3. Red meat: Consuming red meat in large amount has been linked to an increased risk of developing high blood pressure.

4. Sugary beverages: Sugary beverages like juice and soda can cause weight gain and high blood pressure.

Herbs & Supplements for High Blood Pressure

Supplements and herbs may also assist lower blood pressure levels in addition to dietary modifications. These consist of:

1. Omega-3 fatty acids: Fish oil supplements and fatty fish like salmon and tuna include omega-3 fatty acids that help decrease blood pressure.

2. Coenzyme Q10: Also known as CoQ10, this antioxidant is a naturally occurring substance that aids in lowering blood pressure.

3. Garlic: Garlic supplements improve blood flow and dilate blood arteries, which lower blood pressure levels.

4. Hibiscus: Studies have demonstrated a moderate blood pressure-reducing benefit of hibiscus tea.

5. Magnesium: By relaxing blood arteries, magnesium supplements can lower blood pressure levels.

CHAPTER 5

Blood Pressure-Lowering Exercise

While there are a number of treatments for hypertension, including prescription drugs and dietary adjustments, regular exercise is one of the best ways to regulate blood pressure.

Advantages Of Exercise For Lowering Blood Pressure

Blood pressure has been demonstrated to benefit from exercise in a number of ways.

1. It aid in the reduction of both systolic and diastolic blood pressure. This enables the heart to pump blood through the body more effectively since exercise strengthens the heart. As a result, there is less pressure exerted on the artery walls, which might result in a drop in blood pressure.

2. Exercise can enhance general cardiovascular health in addition to decreasing blood pressure. This includes

lowering the risk of cardiovascular disease, stroke, and other related illnesses.

3. Another key aspect of blood pressure control is weight loss, which can also be aided by exercise. Losing weight through exercise can help those who are overweight or obese lower their blood pressure since they are more likely to have high blood pressure.

Exercises to Control Blood Pressure

There are numerous forms of exercise that can lower blood pressure. These consist of:

1. Aerobic exercise: Also referred to as cardio, aerobic exercise is any form of physical activity that increases heart rate and causes deeper breathing. This include exercises like cycling, swimming, dancing, walking, and jogging. At least 30 minutes of moderate exercise should be done on most days of the week.

2. Yoga: Yoga is a form of physical activity that incorporates breathing exercises, meditation, and physical postures. It has been demonstrated to offer several health

advantages, including lowering blood pressure. On most days of the week, try to practice yoga for at least 30 minutes.

3. High-intensity interval training (HIIT): HIIT is an exercise technique that alternates brief bursts of vigorous activity with rest or low-intensity exercise.

It's been proven to be an effective way to improve cardiovascular health and lower blood pressure. strive for two to three workouts per week, with a minimum of one day of rest between each session.

Exercise Duration and Frequency

Exercise must be done consistently to keep blood pressure under control. Choose whether you wish to exercise for 75 minutes at a vigorous intensity or 150 minutes at a moderate intensity per week.

This might also be split up into multiple smaller time chunks throughout the day. Along with aerobic exercise, your workout schedule should include resistance training and yoga.

 Aim for a minimum of two to three workouts of resistance training per week, and spend at least 30 minutes each day of the week practicing yoga.

Precautions for Exercising with High Blood Pressure

Exercise helps lower blood pressure, but you should exercise cautiously if you already have high blood pressure. The following details need to be kept in mind:

1. Begin slowly: It's vital to start softly and increase your intensity over time if you're new to fitness or haven't worked out in a while. This will help you avoid injury and overexertion.

2. Check your blood pressure: If you have high blood pressure, it's a good idea to check it both before and after exercise. This can assist you in determining how your body responds to exercise and whether or not your blood pressure is within a healthy level.

3. Avoid activities that raise blood pressure: Some exercises, such as strenuous weightlifting or those that

require prolonged breath holding, can actually raise blood pressure.

4. Drink lots of water: If you have high blood pressure, it's extremely important to drink lots of water while exercising. Drink plenty of water before, during, and after exercise, as dehydration can cause blood pressure to rise.

5. Recognize the warning indications: Recognize warning indicators including dizziness, shortness of breath, or chest pain. Stop working out right away and get medical help if you encounter any of these symptoms.

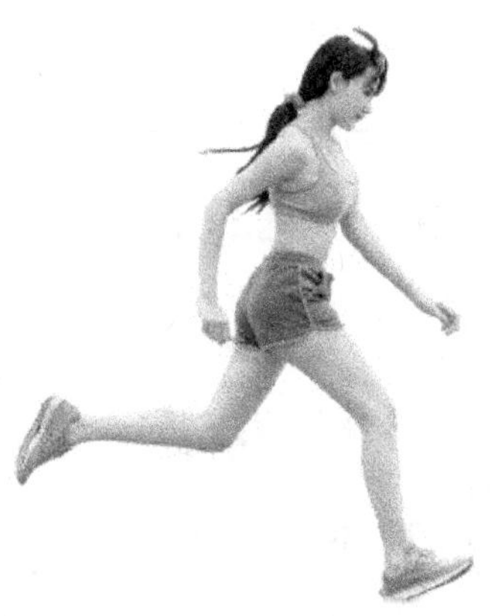

CHAPTER 6

Stress Management for Blood Pressure Control

Stress is a natural part of life. When it persists and is not handled, it can have detrimental impacts on our health, which may lead to high blood pressure.

High blood pressure is a major contributor to stroke, heart disease, and other grave health issues. Stress management helps to regulate blood pressure and lower the risk of certain health issues.

Stress and Blood Pressure

Stress triggers the "fight or flight" reaction in our bodies, which causes the flow of hormonal substances like cortisol and adrenaline.

This reaction is intended to assist us in coping with immediate stressors, such as fleeing from a predator or attending to an urgent situation. These hormones, however, can have detrimental impacts on our health, like raising blood pressure, when stress becomes persistent.

When we are stressed, our heart rate and breathing rate increase, our muscles strain, and our blood vessels constrict. Blood pressure rises as a result of this.

If stress is not successfully controlled over time, this rise in blood pressure may become chronic and result in hypertension.

Stress Management Techniques

The good news is that there are numerous stress management techniques, such as:

1. Exercise: Regular physical activity is a great way to relieve stress and lower blood pressure. Exercise produces endorphins, which are organic mood enhancers that can help reduce anxiety. It also supports cardiovascular health, which can help lower blood pressure.

2. Deep Breathing: Deep breathing help to reduce stress by relaxing the muscles and slowing down heart rates. Sit or lie down in a calm environment. With eyes closed, take

some few deep breaths in through the nostrils and out through the mouth.

3. Progressive Muscle Relaxation: In this method, each muscle group in your body is tensed before being gradually relaxed. This may aid in easing tension in the muscles and encouraging relaxation, which may lessen stress and lower blood pressure.

4. Cognitive Behavioral Therapy (CBT): CBT is a form of talk therapy that can assist you in recognizing the harmful attitudes and conduct that fuel stress and anxiety. CBT can assist in modifying these tendencies to lessen stress and enhance mental wellness.

Steps For CBT At Home

1. Write down self-affirmations to combat negative thoughts.

Once you've identified where your negative ideas are coming from, you may write a self-statement to combat each thought and then continue this process. You'll eventually find that you're thinking more positive ideas than negative ones.

2. Recognize the issue and consider potential remedies.

Talking to someone and keeping a journal can help you identify the source of your problem. You can start by outlining the problems and thinking of a workable solution.

3. Look for new opportunities to think positively.

Whenever you visit a place and all you can see are the things you detest, attempt to identify at least five positive aspects of the location. This will encourage you to think favorably about the location rather than negatively, which could cause stress.

4. Reflect on the best moment of each day before bed.

As soon as your day is over, make sure to record the highlights in your journal. Your mind will build new, positive associations and new neural pathways by recording, registering, and sharing good thoughts.

5. Accept setbacks as a necessary component of living a healthy life.

You must embrace disappointments as a normal part of life if you want to advance in life. Devastation is a valid emotion because it aids in getting through difficult circumstances.

Additionally, you can make a note of the event, the lesson you learned from it, and some resolutions for the future. This will assist you in moving forward with your life.

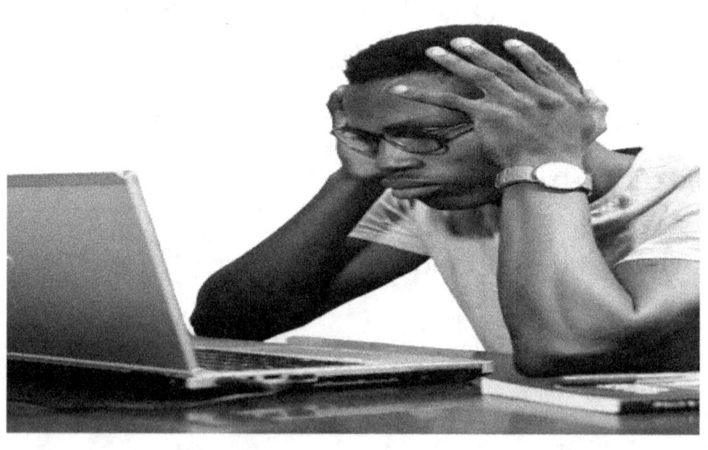

CHAPTER 7

Getting Enough Sleep to Manage Blood Pressure

It is critical for those who are trying to reduce their blood pressure to get enough sleep as it is an important component of maintaining good health. According to research, lack of sleep can contribute to a variety of health issues, including hypertension.

The significance of sleep for controlling blood pressure

Sleep is crucial for blood pressure regulation. Our bodies undergo a process of rejuvenation and repair when we sleep. Our blood pressure drops and our heart rate slows, letting our bodies relax and recover from the events of the day.

But when we are denied enough rest, our bodies are unable to go through this crucial process, which can cause high blood pressure.

According to studies, those who sleep only a few hours a night are more likely to acquire hypertension than those who enjoy a full night's rest. Additionally, studies have linked a higher risk of hypertension to poor sleep quality.

How Much Sleep Is Required for Blood Pressure Control?

The quantity of sleep required for blood pressure control varies from person to person, although most individuals need seven to nine hours of sleep every night. However, quality of sleep is just as crucial as quantity when it comes to health.

High blood pressure and sleep apnea

Breathing interruptions while sleeping are a typical feature of sleep apnea. People who have sleep apnea frequently snore, gasp, or choke while they sleep, which can interfere with their quality of sleep and raise their blood pressure.

According to research, sleep apnea increases the risk of developing hypertension. Research has shown that persons with sleep apnea have a threefold increased risk of hypertension compared to those without the disorder. This is because sleep apnea lowers oxygen levels, which can raise blood pressure.

Factors that lead to obstructive sleep apnea

Several factors have been identified by doctors as contributing to obstructive sleep apnea. These consist of:

1. Being at least 40 years old

2. Overweight

3. Having a history of sleep apnea in the family

4. Excessive intake of alcohol

5. Large overbite

6. Large tongue

7. Smoking

8. Having a tiny jaw

Home remedy for sleep apnea

1. Exercise to reduce overweight

2. Include yoga in your routine

3. Sleep on your side

4. Avoid alcohol before bedtime

5. Use a humidifier

How to Sleep Better

If you struggle to get enough sleep, there are a few things you may do to improve the quality of your sleep. Here are some suggestions for obtaining more sleep:

1. Maintain a consistent sleeping routine. Set a consistent bedtime and wake-up time.

2. Make your surroundings sleep-friendly. Use comfy bedding in a cool, calm, and dark bedroom.

3. Limit coffee and alcohol consumption before bed. Both of these can reduce the quality of sleep and make it more difficult to fall asleep.

4. Exercise frequently. Exercise can lower the chances of hypertension and enhance sleep quality.

5. Work on your relaxation skills. Deep breathing, yoga, and meditation are some methods that can help you relax and have a better night's sleep.

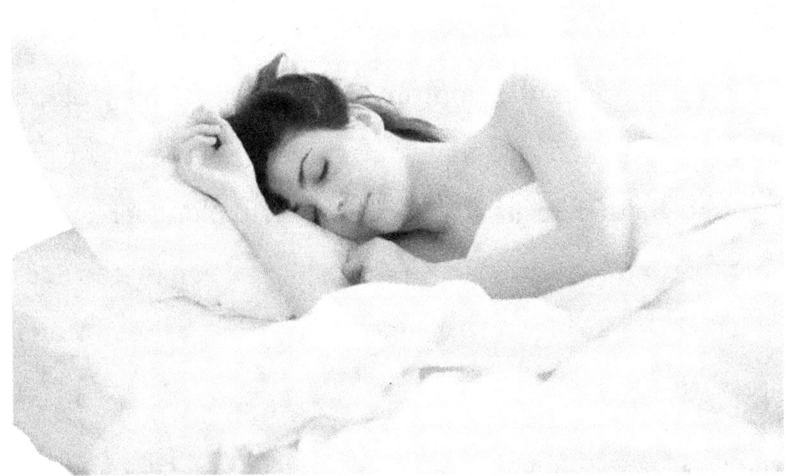

CHAPTER 8

Quitting Smoking for Blood Pressure Control

Smoking is a significant risk factor for high blood pressure. In this section, we will discuss the effects of smoking on blood pressure, the benefits of quitting smoking for blood pressure control, strategies for quitting smoking, and resources for smokers who want to quit.

Effects of Smoking on Blood Pressure

Smoking is a popular contributory factor for high blood pressure. Smokers' blood vessels narrow as a result of the nicotine in their cigarettes, raising their blood pressure. Smoke from cigarettes also contains carbon monoxide, which lowers blood oxygen levels and raises blood pressure.

The effects of smoking a cigarette can linger for up to an hour. Long-term smoking can also affect the lining of blood vessels, making it less flexible and more likely to harden and constrict.

Smoking not only raises blood pressure but also lessens the efficiency of blood pressure drugs. This indicates that smoke addicts with hypertension may require higher dosages of medicine to manage their blood pressure than nonsmokers.

Benefits of Quitting Smoking for Blood Pressure Control

Quitting smoking offers various health benefits, including decreased blood pressure. After quitting smoking, the blood pressure of an individual starts to fall within just 20 minutes.

Blood flow increases within two to three months, and blood pressure might fall by up to ten points. After giving up smoking, the chance of developing heart disease is cut in half within a year.

Additionally, quitting smoking increases the efficiency of blood pressure drugs. The blood pressure-lowering effects of drugs can be efficiently controlled when nicotine's effects are absent.

This suggests that those who give up smoking might be able to take less medicine to manage their blood pressure, lowering the risk of negative effects.

There are other advantages to quitting smoking for cardiovascular health. It can lessen the risk of peripheral artery disease, heart disease, and stroke. Additionally, it can enhance lung health and lower the danger of respiratory infections.

Strategies for Quitting Smoking

Smokers who want to stop often find it difficult, but there are various methods and services accessible to them.

1. Nicotine Replacement Therapy (NRT): NRT is a category of medication that delivers nicotine to the body without the toxic substances contained in cigarettes. NRT helps

lessen the cravings and withdrawal symptoms related to quitting smoking.

2. Prescription Drugs: Several prescription drugs, including bupropion and varenicline, can aid smokers in quitting. These drugs operate by lessening withdrawal symptoms and cravings.

3. Behavioral Support: Providing behavioral support can assist smokers in creating coping mechanisms for cravings and feelings of withdrawal. This can be online support groups, group therapy, or individual counseling.

4. Combination therapy: Combining NRT, prescription drugs, and behavioral support can increase effectiveness.

5. Cold Turkey: Some individuals who smoke prefer to give up the habit completely on their own, without the help of any pharmaceutical or behavioral therapy.

This approach is referred to as "cold turkey." It is feasible to stop smoking with this method, although it can be difficult.

Resources for Smokers Who Want to Quit

There are numerous resources available to assist smokers in giving up, including:

1. Quitlines: This is a telephone-based counseling program that offers help and direction to smokers who want to give up smoking. The National Quitline (1-800-QUIT-NOW) in the US offers free information and counseling to smokers who wish to give up.

2. Online Support: Numerous online services assist smokers in quitting, like websites, forums, and apps. These resources can offer advice, encouragement, and methods for quitting smoking.

3. Nicotine Replacement Therapy (NRT) Products: Most pharmacies sell NRT items over the counter, including patches, gum, lozenges, and inhalers. These goods can lessen the cravings and withdrawal symptoms that come with quitting smoking.

CHAPTER 9

Limiting Alcohol Intake for Blood Pressure Control

In many cultures, drinking alcohol is largely accepted as a social norm, yet if not done so in moderation, it can be harmful to our health.

One of such health concern is the impact of alcohol on blood pressure. Therefore, it is essential to limit alcohol intake to control blood pressure levels and maintain overall health.

Alcohol's Effects on Blood Pressure

A "spike" in blood pressure can occur as a result of drinking alcohol. This increase happens because drinking alcohol relaxes blood arteries and improves blood flow.

However, persistent hypertension can develop over time as a result of excessive alcohol use. When blood pressure is consistently elevated over an extended period, it becomes chronic hypertension.

According to studies, drinking more alcohol increases the likelihood of having hypertension. For instance, drinking excessive amounts of alcohol (defined as having a minimum of three drinks per day) can boost the risk of hypertension by as much as 70%.

Furthermore, alcohol can interfere with hypertension drugs, reducing their effectiveness.

Alcohol Consumption Limits for Blood Pressure Control

Moderation is important when drinking alcohol. According to the American Heart Association, women should consume no more than one drink per day of alcohol, while men should limit their consumption to two drinks per day.

It's vital to note that this advice only applies to typical alcoholic beverages, which are defined as:

- A 12-ounce beer with a 5% alcohol content

- 5 ounces of wine with a 12% alcohol content

- 1.5 ounces of 40% alcohol by volume distilled spirits

When figuring out what amounts of alcohol are safe to consume, it's also crucial to take into account personal aspects like age, weight, and general health.

The consumption of alcohol may need to be further restricted in certain groups, such as older adults and people with pre-existing medical issues.

Tips for Limiting Alcohol Consumption

There are many suggestions you may use to cut down on your consumption and lower your blood pressure if you discover that you are drinking more alcohol than is considered to be safe. These consist of:

1. Establish a limit. Choose the amount of alcohol you would like to consume each day and adhere to it. At first, this could seem difficult, but with experience, it gets simpler.

2. Monitor your consumption: Keep track of the amount of alcohol you drink each day. This can aid in raising your awareness of your drinking patterns and pointing out areas where you can limit your intake.

3. Consume beverages that are free from alcohol: Drink fruit juice, or water. This helps to cut back on alcohol intake.

4. Maintain a steady pace. Instead of guzzling your drink, sip it slowly. This will increase the enjoyment of your beverage and lower your overall intake.

5. Refrain from binge drinking: Binge drinking is defined as having a minimum of four drinks in two hours for women or greater than five drinks in two hours for men. Binge drinking can induce a sharp increase in blood pressure. Attempt to completely avoid excessive drinking.

6. Seek assistance: If you're having problems controlling your alcohol use on your own, consider asking for assistance from your family, friends, or a medical

professional. They can provide you with the guidance and inspiration you need to limit your alcohol consumption.

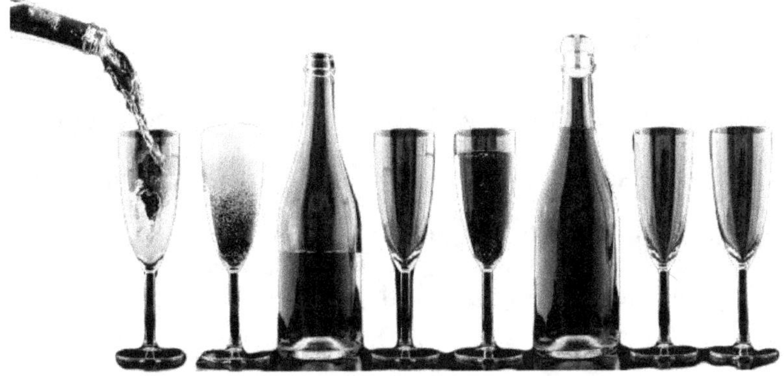

CHAPTER 10

Maintaining a Healthy Weight for Blood Pressure Control

Maintaining a suitable weight is critical for your general well-being, and it is especially vital for blood pressure control. Fortunately, there are several methods for obtaining and keeping a healthy weight that can assist in reducing blood pressure and enhancing general health.

Relationship between Weight and Blood Pressure

The connection between blood pressure and weight is obvious. According to studies, a significant risk factor for high blood pressure is being overweight or obese.

Your heart needs to work harder to circulate blood throughout your body when you are overweight. Your blood pressure could increase as a result of the increased workload.

Additionally, excess weight can cause changes in your body that can contribute to high blood pressure.

Benefits of Losing Weight for Blood Pressure Control

The good news is that losing just a little weight can help to lower blood pressure, cut the risk of heart disease, and prevent other health issues. According to studies, even a small weight loss of 5–10% of your body weight can significantly lower blood pressure.

Weight loss can assist to reduce blood pressure in a variety of ways. The first benefit is that it can lessen the amount of fat and other tissue that your heart needs to pump blood to, thereby reducing the strain on your heart. This can aid in the reduction of systolic and diastolic blood pressure.

Losing weight can also assist to increase insulin sensitivity, which can result in lower insulin levels and less blood vessel constriction. This may aid in enhancing blood flow and bringing down blood pressure.

Finally, lowering weight can help to reduce inflammation in the body, which is a major cause of hypertension and other health problems. Lowering inflammation can improve blood vessel health and minimize your risk of heart attack and stroke.

Strategies for Maintaining a Healthy Weight

There are several methods you can use to help you reach and keep a healthy weight. These consist of:

1. Consume a healthy diet: Consumption of healthy food is one of the most important factors in achieving and sustaining a healthy weight. Consume a variety of veggies, whole grains, fruits, lean meats, and healthy fats as your primary food groups. Avoid processed foods, sugary beverages, and other unhealthy items that may result in weight gain.

2. Exercise regularly: Regular exercise is necessary to maintain a healthy weight and regulate blood pressure. Try to engage in moderate activity most days of the week

for at least 30 minutes. This can involve activities like vigorous walking, dancing, swimming, and cycling.

3. Get enough rest: Sleep is necessary for maintaining a healthy weight. strive for seven to eight hours of sleep each night to help with hormone regulation that affects hunger and metabolism.

4. Control your stress: Prolonged tension can lead to weight gain and high blood pressure. Engage in stress-relieving hobbies like yoga, meditation, or deep breathing.

5. Keep an eye on your weight: Maintaining a regular weight-monitoring routine can help you stay on track and make necessary modifications.

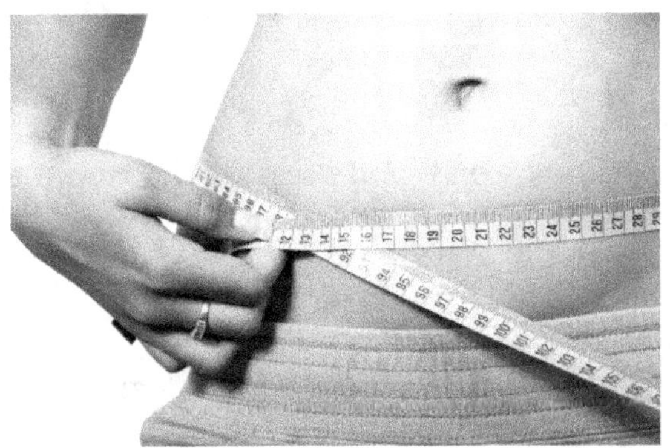

CHAPTER 11

Checking Your Blood Pressure at Home

Blood pressure is an important measure of cardiovascular health. Any anomalies in blood pressure may be a sign of underlying medical issues because it measures the force of blood flowing through the arteries.

Stroke, cardiovascular disease, and renal failure are all significantly increased risks of hypertension. Regular blood pressure tests are a standard component of the majority of medical examinations because of how important it is to track blood pressure.

The Importance of Home Blood Pressure Monitoring

Keeping close tabs on blood pressure measurements over time is easy and reliable with home blood pressure monitors. Home readings for blood pressure are collected in comfortable settings and can give a clearer indication of a person's general blood pressure history than measurements made in a clinic, which are done under controlled circumstances and may be impacted by things like tension and anxiety.

Furthermore, monitoring one's blood pressure at home can give medical experts useful data that can inform treatment choices. People who monitor their blood pressure levels at home can spot any changes in it and adapt their lifestyles or, if necessary, seek medical assistance.

Periodic observation at home can also assist people with hypertension in understanding the effects of their medications and modifying their dosages or treatment programs as needed.

Types of Home Blood Pressure Monitors

There are two varieties of home blood pressure monitors available.

1. The most popular and reliable form of home blood pressure monitor is an upper arm monitor, which is more

precise than a wrist monitor. They consist of an inflatable cuff that is put over the upper arm to take blood pressure readings.

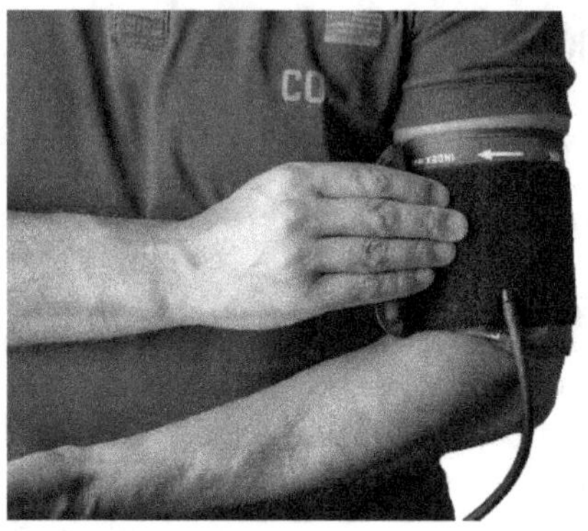

2. In contrast, wrist monitors are more compact than upper arm monitors but might not give readings that are precise. They employ a sensor to detect blood pressure and are fastened on the wrist.

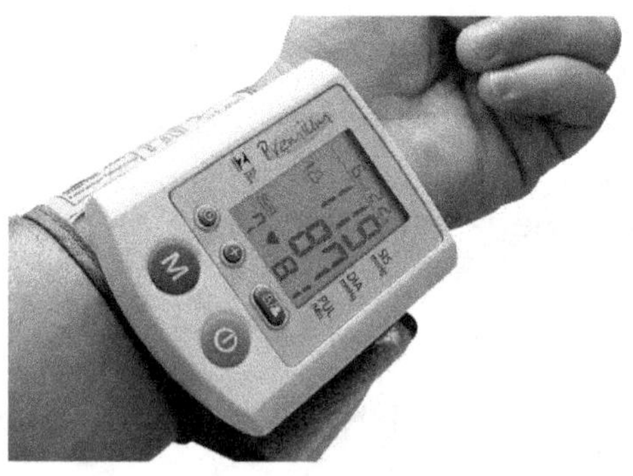

How to Monitor Blood Pressure Correctly at Home

People should closely adhere to the instructions that came with their blood pressure devices to obtain reliable readings of their blood pressure at home. Here are some broad pointers for precise home blood pressure tracking:

1. Before taking a reading, sit calmly for a minimum of five minutes.

2. Ensure that the cuff is snugly secured around the wrist or upper arm.

3. Take two or three readings spaced one minute apart. Then, note the average of the measurements.

4. Take readings every day at the same time, preferably before taking any medications.

5. Spend at least 30 minutes without coffee, cigarettes, or activity before getting a reading.

6. Try not to talk or cross your legs while being measured.

CHAPTER 12

Relationships that help lower blood pressure

According to research, maintaining healthy blood pressure can be influenced favorably by profound connections with others and social ties.

Understanding the function of social support can help develop more thorough strategies for controlling blood pressure while highlighting the importance of human connection and a holistic view of well-being.

The Importance of Social Support in Blood Pressure Management

Social support is the term used to describe the psychological, practical, and educational help given by others. It can originate from a variety of places, including loved ones, peers, or support groups.

The following are some methods that social interaction can aid with blood pressure regulation:

1. Encouragement and Motivation: People with hypertension who have supportive relationships may find it easier to stick to their medications. Individuals are inclined to stick to their medication schedule, maintain a nutritious meal plan, and participate in frequent exercise when they recognize that they can rely on someone.

2. Stress management: High blood pressure is frequently brought on by stress. Supportive connections can help people manage stress by lending a listening ear, delivering practical guidance, or offering a respite from difficult events.

3. Information and Resources: close companions can offer helpful guidance and materials for managing blood pressure, such as wholesome foods, advice on exercising, or details on nearby support groups.

4. Accountability: Supportive connections can make people responsible for controlling their blood pressure. People may be inspired to adhere to their medication regimen if they realize that a person is monitoring their progress.

Building Supportive Relationships

While social support might help with hypertension treatment, not every individual has a network of support. Here are some pointers for developing sustaining relationships:

1. Become a member of a support group: Support networks are a terrific method to meet people going through comparable circumstances. They can give you a sense of belonging, emotional support, and useful tips for controlling your blood pressure. Much peer support is provided online, making them open to people who couldn't find local options.

2. Volunteer: Volunteering can offer chances to make new friends and develop connections based on common interests. Additionally, it can give a sense of satisfaction and purpose, which is good for general well-being.

3. Engage in Social Activities: Social activities, like embracing a sports team, enrolling in a class, or going to a

local event, can help you discover new individuals and develop relationships.

4. Reach Out to Family and Friends: Try to stay in touch with your family and friends regularly if they are supportive of you. Make phone calls, arrange a coffee date, or engage in activities together.

The Role of Family and Friends in Blood Pressure Control

Friends and acquaintances can be quite important in managing hypertension. Here are several methods in which they could assist:

1. Encourage Healthy Habits: close companions can support persons who have high blood pressure by encouraging healthy habits including eating a nutritious diet, exercising frequently, and abstaining from cigarette use and binge drinking.

2. Offer Useful Help: Family members and friends can offer useful help, such as food shopping, the cooking of meals, or transportation to doctor's visits.

3. Provide Emotional Support: Supporting someone emotionally by listening to them and encouraging them can help people with hypertension handle stress and maintain their motivation to follow their treatment plan.

4. Participate in the Treatment Plan: Family members and friends can assist in the course of treatment by going with the patient to appointments, assisting to check blood pressure, and encouraging the patient to take their prescribed drugs.

Support Groups and Additional Resources for High Blood Pressure Patients

Patients with high blood pressure have access to a variety of resources, such as support groups and other tools. Here are a few examples:

1. American Heart Association (AHA): The AHA is a charitable organization that offers services for people with hypertension, including informational resources, peer support, and lifestyle control programs.

2. National High Blood Pressure Education Program (NHBPEP): The American Heart Association and the National Institutes of Health worked together to develop this program. The program provides resources, therapeutic guidelines, and educational materials for healthcare professionals and persons with hypertension.

3. Local Support Groups: You can connect with people who may be going through comparable experiences by joining local support groups. Online support networks are open to the public, making them available to people who might not have a chance to visit them locally.

4. Hypertension Apps: Many apps can assist individuals with monitoring their blood pressure, managing their medications, and managing their lifestyles. Examples include MyPlate, MyFitnessPal, and Blood Pressure Companion.

5. Healthcare Professionals: Qualified dietitians, primary care doctors, and cardiologists can all offer advice and assistance for controlling hypertension.

CHAPTER 13

Nutrition and Blood Pressure Control

Blood pressure management is significantly influenced by nutrition. The degree of blood pressure and general cardiovascular health can be directly impacted by specific food decisions.

Nutritional Deficiencies and High Blood Pressure

Deficiencies in some nutrients might influence elevated blood pressure. For instance, the body's capacity to control blood pressure might be hampered by insufficient consumption of calcium, potassium, magnesium, and vitamin D.

Magnesium is a necessary mineral that regulates blood pressure, heartbeat, muscle and neuron function, and many other biological processes. Insufficient amounts of magnesium have been linked in studies to high hypertension and a higher risk of heart disease.

Another necessary element for healthy bones, dental structure, and muscular growth is calcium. It assists in controlling blood pressure by controlling the compression and relaxation of blood vessels. According to several research, low calcium intake is associated with high blood pressure.

Vitamin D, often referred to as sunshine's vitamin, is essential for strong bones and a robust immune system. Lack of vitamin D has been linked to a higher risk of hypertension.

It is crucial to eat nutritious meals full of nutrient-dense foods like veggies, whole grain foods, fruits, lean meats, and nutritious fats to avoid nutrient shortages that can increase blood pressure.

Sodium and High Blood Pressure

Sodium, a mineral found in salt, is an essential component for maintaining fluid balance, neuron activity, and muscle contraction. But eating too much sodium can increase blood pressure by increasing the volume of blood flowing through the body, which puts greater strain on the heart.

It is critical to minimize the eating of processed foods, quick foods, and snacks that are salty in order to lower sodium intake. Instead, choose fresh, healthy foods and season dishes with salt-free spice blends and seasonings.

Potassium and High Blood Pressure

The American Heart Association advises getting 4,700 mg or more of potassium from dietary sources each day. Unfortunately, research indicates that a large number of Americans fall short of this requirement, with an estimated daily average consumption of 2,500–3,000 mg.

It is crucial to eat different kinds of veggies, fruits, and whole grains to improve potassium consumption. A variety of sweet potatoes spinach, bananas, avocados, and beans are a few of the greatest foods to eat when looking for potassium.

CHAPTER 14

Tracking Progress and Maintaining Blood Pressure

Keeping track of blood pressure levels periodically can give important insights into the efficacy of dietary adjustments, medication, and other measures meant to manage hypertension or keep blood pressure levels at a healthy level.

The Importance of Monitoring Progress in Blood Pressure Control

Monitoring blood pressure changes is crucial for blood pressure management. It enables people to keep track of their blood pressure readings and make health-related decisions with knowledge.

Regularly monitoring blood pressure enables people to spot trends and cycles that may have an effect on the level of their blood pressure and to take the necessary steps to manage it.

Monitoring blood pressure changes can also assist people in seeing any early warning signs of prospective health issues. For instance, a sudden rise in blood pressure may call for a prescription adjustment or a modification of lifestyle choices.

Additionally, monitoring progress might keep people inspired to keep up their blood pressure control efforts. A person may be more likely to maintain healthy behaviors and continue taking their medicine as directed if they can see results.

Blood pressure-tracking apps for keeping a journal

Keeping a journal is one efficient technique to monitor your blood pressure's progress. A simple notebook or an in-depth electronic journal both work well for keeping track of blood pressure.

People who keep track of their blood pressure measurements, drugs used, and lifestyle choices might spot patterns and trends that might be affecting their blood pressure levels.

Additionally, there are numerous blood pressure monitoring apps for smartphones and other technological devices. These apps let users log their blood pressure readings and monitor their development over time.

Additionally, some apps provide features like blood pressure graphs, prescription reminders, and lifestyle tracking. Here are a few popular choices:

1. Blood Pressure Companion (iOS): This app enables you to monitor and evaluate your weight, heart rate, and blood pressure readings. To analyze your progress and patterns, it offers simple-to-read graphs and charts. You can also make reports to send to your healthcare physician and schedule medication alerts.

2. My BP Lab (Android): Designed by Samsung and the University of California, San Francisco, this app measures your blood pressure and stress levels using the sensors on your smartphone. You can take part in research activities

and receive individualized comments as well as information based on your readings.

3. Health Mate (iOS, Android): You may monitor different health parameters, including blood pressure, with Withings' Health Mate app. They can automatically link your readings with their blood pressure monitors to get customised advice. You may establish objectives and reminders using the app's user-friendly layout.

4. Heart Habit (iOS): Heart Habit aids in monitoring and managing your cardiovascular and blood pressure wellness. It offers graphs and trends to make your progress over time easier to grasp. You can export your data as well and give it to your physician.

5. iBP Blood Pressure (iOS, Android): This app lets you log and track your blood pressure measurements as well as other health information like weight, prescription information, and notes. It offers thorough reports and graphs to make it easier for you to see your progress and communicate with your healthcare professional.

Staying Motivated for Long-Term Blood Pressure Control

It can be difficult to maintain motivation to manage blood pressure over time. People can utilize a variety of techniques to maintain their motivation and attention on their health-related objectives.

Setting reasonable and realistic goals is a good strategy. Setting manageable, short-term objectives might assist people in maintaining motivation and gaining momentum over time. For instance, a person could start by setting a goal of losing 1-2 pounds every week rather than trying to drop 20 pounds.

Another tactic is to come up with fun methods to make healthy behaviors a part of daily life. People could, for instance, discover a physical activity they enjoy, like dancing, hiking, or swimming, rather than loathing exercise.

Finally, acknowledging accomplishments can serve as a strong motivation. People can increase their confidence and drive to keep up their blood pressure management efforts by acknowledging and appreciating their victories.

CHAPTER 15

Seven-Day Meal Plan For High Blood Pressure Management

Here is a sample menu for a week that will help you manage high blood pressure:

Day 1

Breakfast

Oatmeal with Blueberries and Almond Milk

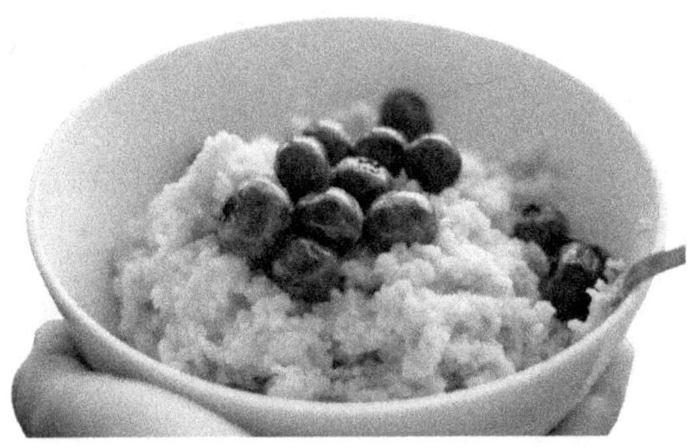

Ingredients

- 1/2 cup rolled oats

- 1 cup unsweetened almond milk

- 1/2 cup blueberries

- 1 tbsp honey (optional)

- Pinch of cinnamon

Preparation

1. In a small saucepan, combine the rolled oats and almond milk and bring to a boil.

2. Cook the oats and allow the mixture to thicken, reduce heat to low and simmer for 5 to 7 minutes, stirring regularly.

3. Add the cinnamon, honey (if using), and blueberries.

4. Serve hot.

Snack

Apple Slices with Almond Butter

Ingredients

- 1 apple, sliced

- 2 tbsp almond butter

Preparation

- Spread the almond butter on the apple slices

- Enjoy!

Lunch

Balsamic Vinaigrette and Grilled Chicken with Spinach and Strawberry Salad

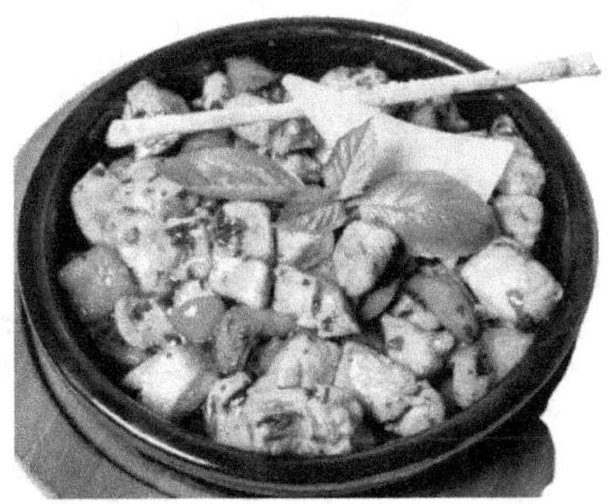

Ingredients

- 2 cups spinach

- 1/2 cup sliced strawberries

- 3 oz grilled chicken breast, sliced

- 1 tbsp balsamic vinegar

- 1 tbsp olive oil

- Salt and pepper, to taste

Preparation

1. Combine the cut strawberries, grilled chicken, and spinach in a big bowl.

2. Combine the olive oil, balsamic vinegar, salt, and pepper in a small bowl.

3. Pour the salad with the dressing, then toss to incorporate.

4. Serve right away.

Snack

Carrots and Hummus

Ingredients

- 1 cup baby carrots

- 1/4 cup hummus

Preparation

Serve the baby carrots with the hummus for dipping.

Dinner

Grilled Salmon with Asparagus and Brown Rice

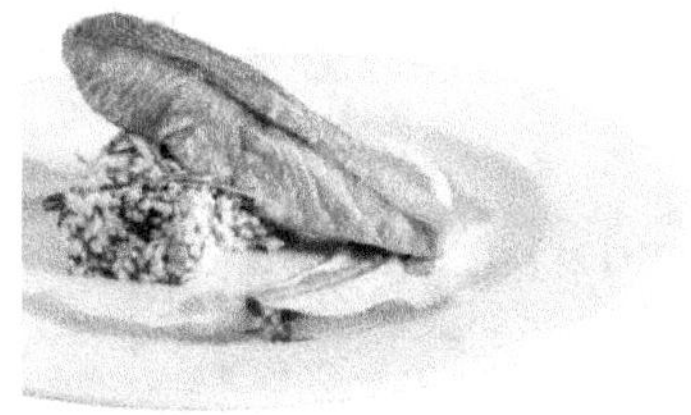

Ingredients

- 4 oz salmon fillet

- 1/2 cup cooked brown rice

- 1/2 cup asparagus spears

- 1 tsp olive oil

- Salt and pepper, to taste

Preparation

1. Heat the grill to a medium-high setting.

2. After coating the salmon fillet with olive oil, season it with salt and pepper.

3. Grill the salmon for four to six minutes on each side.

4. Combine the asparagus spears with salt, pepper, and olive oil.

5. Grill the asparagus until fork-tender, about two to three minutes per side.

6. Include brown rice and grilled asparagus with the grilled fish.

Day 2

Breakfast

Greek Yogurt with Raspberries and Chia Seeds

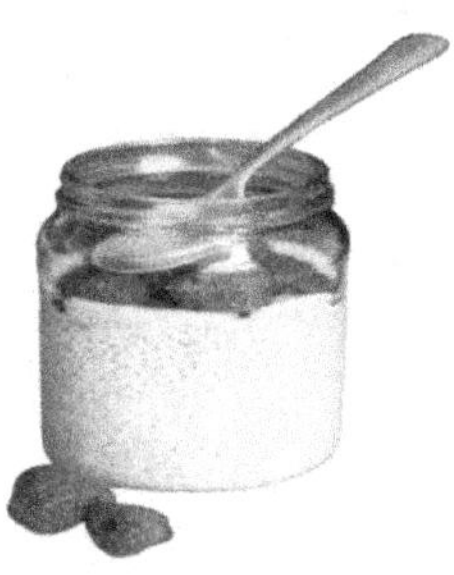

Ingredients

- 1 cup plain Greek yogurt

- 1/2 cup raspberries

- 1 tbsp chia seeds

Preparation

1. In a bowl, mix the Greek yogurt and chia seeds.

2. Top with raspberries.

3. Enjoy!

Snack

Banana with Peanut Butter

Ingredients

- 1 banana

- 1 tbsp natural peanut butter

Preparation

1. Spread the peanut butter on the banana.

2. Enjoy!

Lunch

Whole wheat tortilla with turkey and avocado wrap

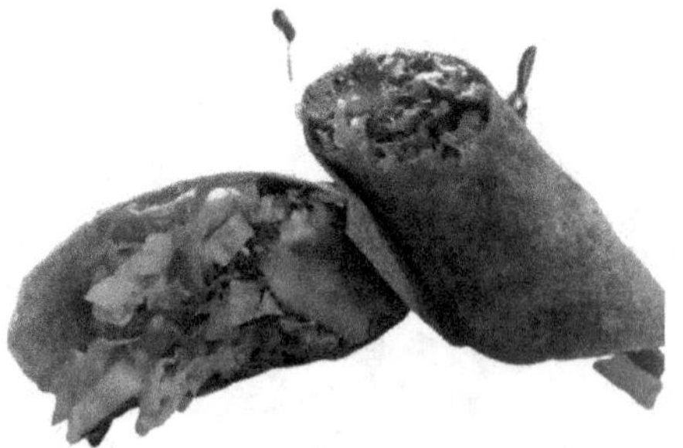

Ingredients

- 3 oz turkey breast, sliced

- 1/4 avocado, sliced

- 1 whole wheat tortilla

- 1/4 cup baby spinach leaves

- 1 tbsp Dijon mustard

- Salt and pepper, to taste

Preparation

1. Lay the whole wheat tortilla on a flat surface.

2. Spread the Dijon mustard on the tortilla.

3. Add the sliced turkey breast, avocado, and baby spinach leaves.

4. Season with salt and pepper.

5. Roll up the tortilla and slice it in half.

6. Serve immediately.

Snack

Edamame

Ingredients

1 cup edamame, cooked and salted

Preparation

1. Serve the edamame in a bowl.

2. Enjoy!

Dinner

Baked Chicken Thighs with Roasted Vegetables

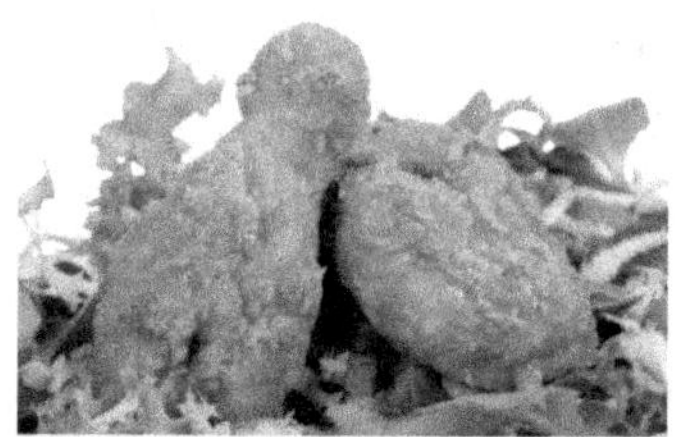

Ingredients

- 2 chicken thighs, bone-in, and skin-on

- 1 cup broccoli florets

- 1 cup sliced bell peppers

- 1/2 cup sliced onion

- 1 tsp olive oil

- Salt and pepper, to taste

Preparation

1. Preheat oven to 400°F.

2. Arrange the chicken thighs on a baking sheet and season with salt and pepper.

3. Roast the chicken for 25-30 minutes, or until cooked through and golden brown.

4. Toss the broccoli florets, bell peppers, and onion with olive oil, salt, and pepper.

5. Add the vegetables to the baking sheet with the chicken and roast for an additional 15-20 minutes, or until tender.

6. Serve the baked chicken thighs with the roasted vegetables.

Day 3

Breakfast

Veggie and Egg Scramble

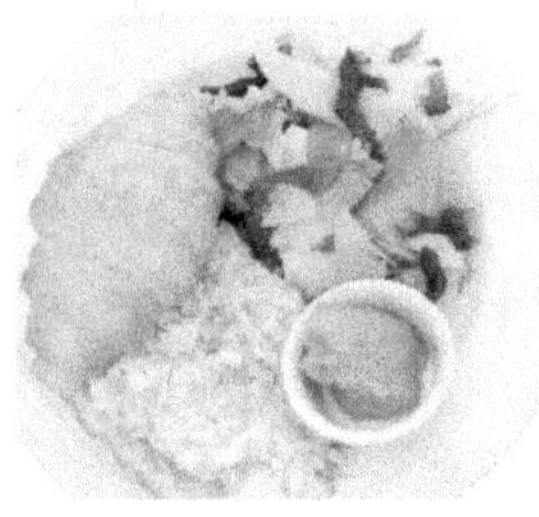

Ingredients

- 2 eggs

- 1/2 cup sliced bell peppers

- 1/2 cup sliced mushrooms

- 1/4 cup diced onion

- 1 tsp olive oil

- Salt and pepper to taste

Preparation

1. Whisk the eggs in a mixing dish and season with salt and pepper.

2. Heat the olive oil in a nonstick skillet over medium heat.

3. Add the diced onion, mushrooms, and bell pepper slices to the skillet and cook for 3–4 minutes, or until they are cooked.

4. Add the whisked eggs to the skillet of veggies and scramble them until they are fully cooked.

5. Serve hot.

Snack

Orange Slices

Ingredients

1 orange, peeled and sliced

Preparation

1. Serve the orange slices in a bowl.

2. Enjoy!

Lunch

Quinoa Salad with Grilled Shrimp and Lemon Vinaigrette

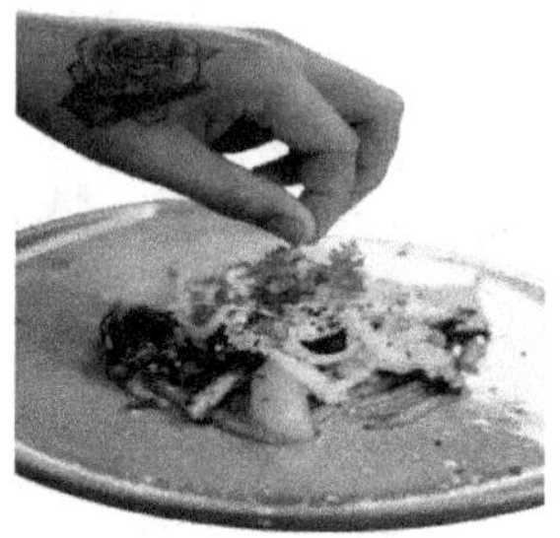

Ingredients

- 1 cup cooked quinoa

- 3 oz grilled shrimp

- 1/2 cup cherry tomatoes, halved

- 1/4 cup diced cucumber

- 1 tbsp lemon juice

- 1 tbsp olive oil

- Salt and pepper to taste

Preparation

1. Mix the cooked quinoa, grilled shrimp, cherry tomatoes, and diced cucumber in a large bowl.

2. Whisk together the lemon juice, olive oil, salt, and pepper to make the vinaigrette in a small bowl.

3. Drizzle the vinaigrette over the quinoa salad and toss to combine.

4. Serve immediately.

Snack

Cottage Cheese with Pineapple Chunks

Ingredients

- 1/2 cup cottage cheese

- 1/2 cup pineapple chunks

Preparation

1. Serve the cottage cheese in a bowl.

2. Top with pineapple chunks.

3. Enjoy!

Dinner

Green beans and sweet potatoes with baked salmon

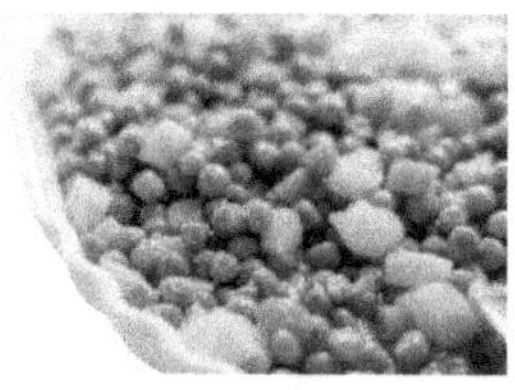

Ingredients

- 4 oz salmon fillet

- 1 medium sweet potato, peeled and diced

- 1 cup green beans, trimmed

- 1 tsp olive oil

- Salt and pepper to taste

Preparation

1. Preheat oven to 400°F.

2. Put the salmon fillet on a baking sheet and season with pepper and salt.

3. Toss the diced sweet potato and green beans with olive oil, salt, and pepper.

4. Add the sweet potato and green beans to the baking sheet with the salmon.

5. Roast for 15-20 minutes, or until the salmon is cooked through and the sweet potato is tender.

6. Serve immediately.

Day 4

Breakfast

Greek Yogurt with Berries and Almonds

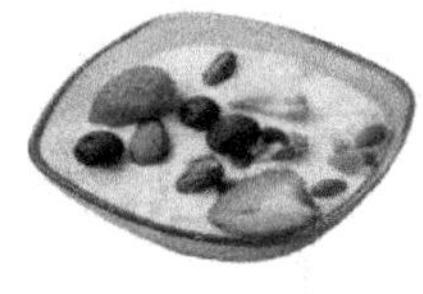

Ingredients

- 1/2 cup plain Greek yogurt

- 1/2 cup mixed berries

- 1 tbsp sliced almonds

Preparation

1. Serve the Greek yogurt in a bowl.

2. Top with mixed berries and sliced almonds.

3. Enjoy!

Snack

Apple Slices with Peanut Butter

Ingredients

- 1 apple, sliced

- 1 tbsp peanut butter

Preparation

1. Spread peanut butter on apple slices.

2. Enjoy!

Lunch

Turkey and Hummus Wrap

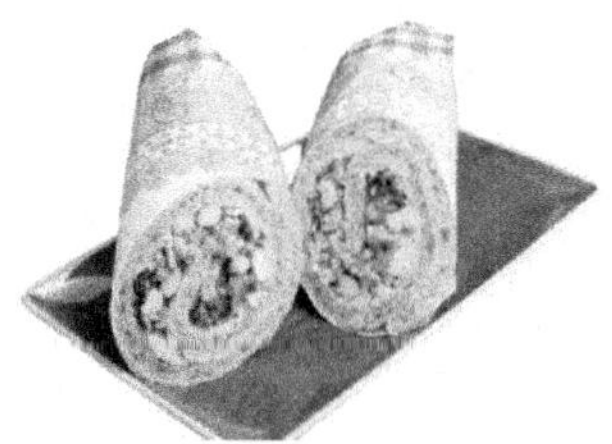

Ingredients

- 1 whole wheat tortilla

- 3 oz sliced turkey breast

- 2 tbsp hummus

- 1/4 cup shredded carrots

- 1/4 cup baby spinach leaves

- Salt and pepper to taste

Preparation

1. Place the tortilla flat on a plate.

2. Spread the hummus on the tortilla.

3. Add the sliced turkey breast, shredded carrots, and baby spinach leaves.

4. Season with salt and pepper.

5. Roll up the tortilla and slice it in half.

6. Serve immediately.

Snack

Carrot Sticks with Hummus

Ingredients

- 1 cup carrot sticks

- 2 tbsp hummus

Preparation

1. Serve the carrot sticks in a bowl.

2. Serve the hummus in a separate bowl for dipping.

3. Enjoy!

Dinner

Beef Stir-Fry with Brown Rice

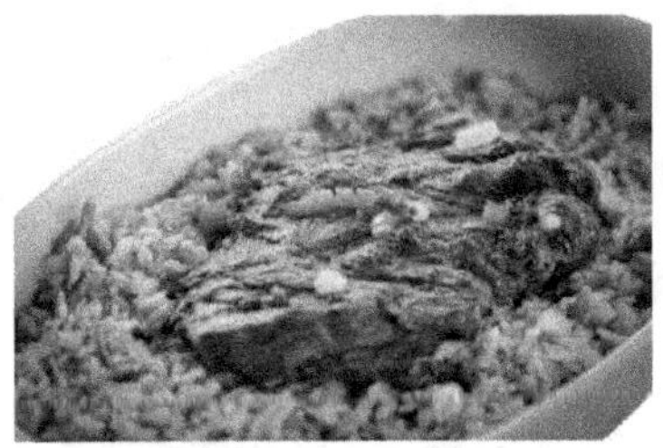

Ingredients

- 4 oz lean beef, sliced

- 1 cup mixed stir-fried vegetables (broccoli, carrots, bell peppers)

- 1/2 cup cooked brown rice

- 1 tsp olive oil

- 2 tbsp low-sodium soy sauce

- 1/4 tsp ground ginger

Preparation

1. Using a skillet, heat the olive oil over medium-high heat.

2. Add the sliced beef and stir-fry for 2-3 minutes, or until browned.

3. Add the mixed vegetables to the skillet and stir-fry for a further 3–4 minutes, or until they are soft.

4. Whisk together the soy sauce and ground ginger in a small bowl.

5. Add the cooked brown rice to the skillet and toss to mix with the beef and vegetables.

6. Drizzle the soy sauce mixture over the stir-fry and toss to coat.

7. Serve immediately.

Day 5

Breakfast

Oatmeal with Blueberries and Walnuts

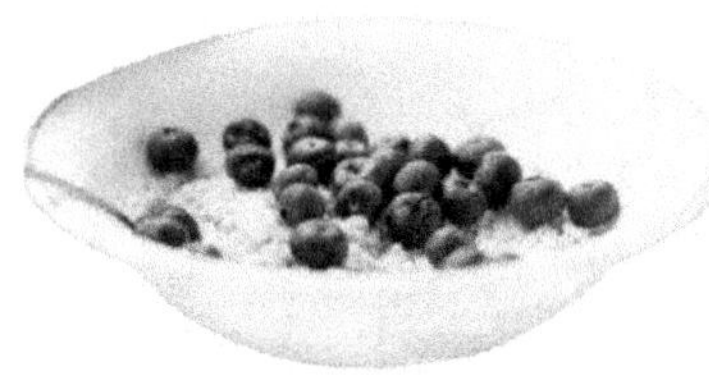

Ingredients

- 1/2 cup rolled oats

- 1 cup water

- 1/4 cup blueberries

- 1 tbsp chopped walnuts

Preparation

1. In a small saucepan, bring the rolled oats and water to a boil.

2. Lower the heat to a simmer and cook the oats for 5 to 7 minutes, or until they are soft and the water has been absorbed.

3. Serve the oatmeal in a bowl.

4. Top with blueberries and chopped walnuts.

5. Enjoy!

Snack

Yogurt and Granola

Ingredients

- 1/2 cup plain low-fat yogurt

- 1/4 cup granola

Preparation

1. Serve the yogurt in a bowl.

2. Top with granola.

3. Enjoy!

Lunch

Grilled Chicken Salad with Avocado and Tomatoes

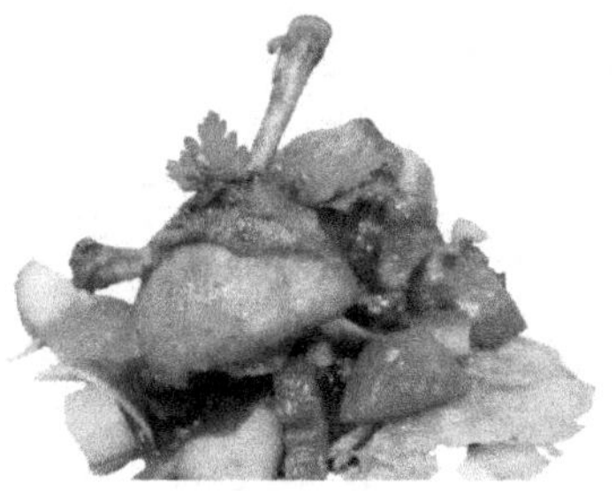

Ingredients

- 3 oz grilled chicken breast

- 2 cups mixed salad greens

- 1/2 avocado, sliced

- 1/2 cup cherry tomatoes, halved

- 1 tbsp olive oil

- 1 tbsp balsamic vinegar

- Salt and pepper, to taste

Preparation

1. Arrange the mixed salad greens on a plate.

2. Add the sliced avocado and cherry tomatoes.

3. Top with the grilled chicken breast.

4. Whisk the olive oil, balsamic vinegar, salt, and pepper in a small bowl.

5. Drizzle the dressing over the salad.

6. Serve immediately.

Snack

Edamame

Ingredients

1 cup edamame, cooked and shelled

Preparation

1. Serve the cooked and shelled edamame in a bowl.

2. Enjoy!

Dinner

Baked Salmon with Quinoa and Roasted Vegetables

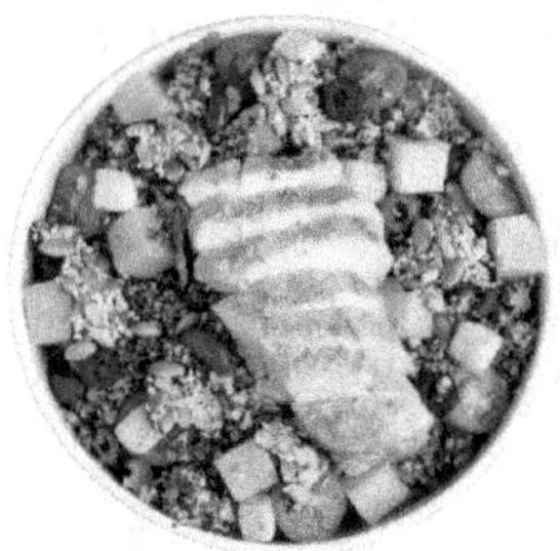

Ingredients

- 4 oz salmon fillet

- 1/2 cup cooked quinoa

- 1 cup mixed roasted vegetables (broccoli, carrots, zucchini)

- 1 tbsp olive oil

- Salt and pepper to taste

Preparation

1. Set the oven's temperature to 400°F (200°C).

2. Put the salmon fillet on a baking sheet.

3. Add a drizzle of olive oil and sprinkle with salt and pepper.

4. Bake the salmon for 10 to 12 minutes, or until it is thoroughly cooked.

5. In a separate baking dish, arrange the mixed roasted vegetables.

6. Drizzle with olive oil and season with salt and pepper.

7. Roast for 15-20 minutes, or until tender.

8. Serve the baked salmon with the cooked quinoa and roasted vegetables.

Breakfast

Whole Wheat Toast and Spinach with Scrambled Eggs

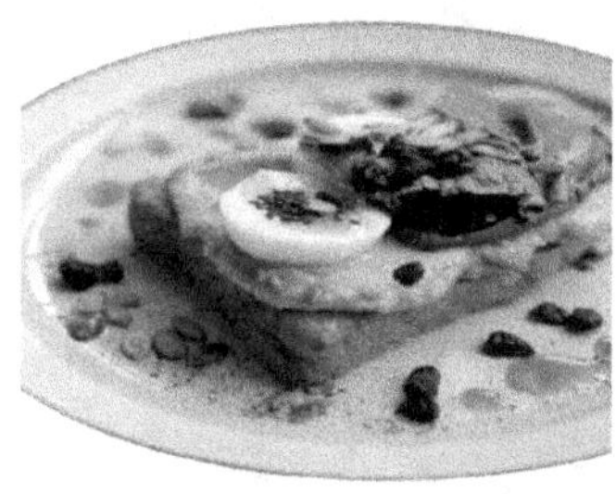

Ingredients

- 2 eggs

- 1/2 cup baby spinach leaves

- 1 slice whole wheat toast

- Salt and pepper, to taste

Preparation

1. Whisk the eggs, baby spinach leaves, salt, and pepper in a small bowl.

2. Preheat a nonstick skillet to medium heat.

3. When the eggs are scrambled and fully cooked, add the egg mixture to the skillet and heat, stirring occasionally.

4. Toast the slice of whole wheat bread.

5. Serve the scrambled eggs with the toasted whole wheat bread.

6. Enjoy!

Snack

Trail Mix

Ingredients

- 1/4 cup mixed nuts (almonds, walnuts, pistachios)

- 1/4 cup dried fruit (raisins, apricots, cranberries)

Preparation

1. Mix the nuts and dried fruit together in a bowl.

2. Enjoy!

Lunch

Tuna Salad Sandwich on Whole Wheat Bread

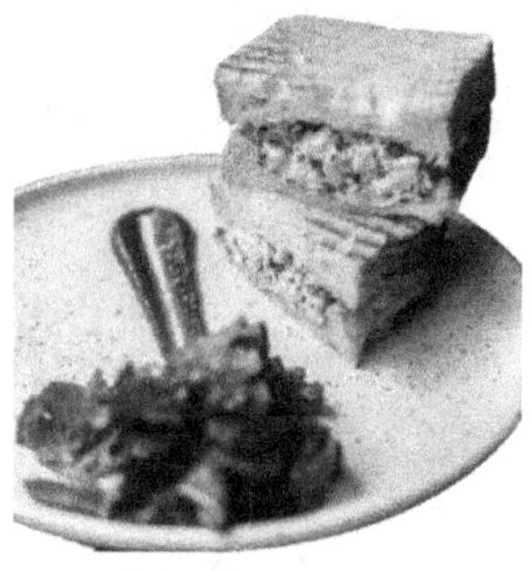

Ingredients

- 1 can tuna in water, drained

- 1 tbsp light mayonnaise

- 1 tbsp chopped celery

- 1 tbsp chopped red onion

- 1 slice whole wheat bread

- Mixed greens, for serving

Preparation

1. Mix the tuna, light mayonnaise, celery, and red onion in a small bowl.

2. Toast the slice of whole wheat bread.

3. Arrange mixed greens on top of the toast.

4. Spoon the tuna salad on top of the mixed greens.

5. Top with another slice of whole wheat bread.

6. Enjoy!

Snack

Sliced Cucumbers with Hummus

Ingredients

- 1 cup sliced cucumbers

- 2 tbsp hummus

Preparation

1. Serve the sliced cucumbers in a bowl.

2. Serve the hummus in a separate bowl for dipping.

3. Enjoy!

Dinner

Brown Rice and Steamed Broccoli with Grilled Chicken

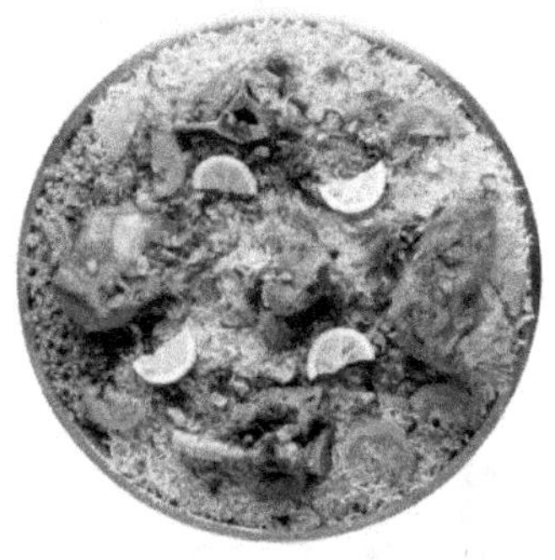

Ingredients

- 4 oz chicken breast

- 1/2 cup cooked brown rice

- 1 cup steamed broccoli

- 1 tbsp olive oil

- Salt and pepper to taste

Preparation

1. Preheat the grill to medium-high heat.

2. Add salt and pepper to the chicken breast.

3. Apply olive oil to the chicken's two sides.

4. Grill the chicken for 6-7 minutes per side, or until cooked through.

5. In a separate pot, cook the brown rice according to the package instructions.

6. In another pot, steam the broccoli for 3-4 minutes, or until tender.

7. Serve the grilled chicken with cooked brown rice and steamed broccoli.

8. Enjoy!

Breakfast

Greek Yogurt with Berries and Almonds

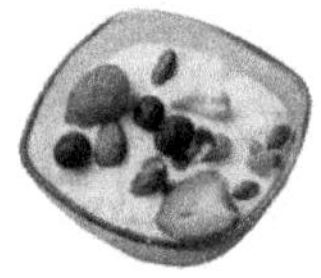

Ingredients

- 1/2 cup plain Greek yogurt

- 1/4 cup mixed berries (blueberries, raspberries, strawberries)

- 1 tbsp slivered almonds

Preparation

1. In a bowl, mix the Greek yogurt and mixed berries.

2. Sprinkle the slivered almonds on top.

3. Enjoy!

Snack

Apple Slices with Peanut Butter

Ingredients

- 1 medium apple, sliced

- 2 tbsp natural peanut butter

Preparation

1. Serve the apple slices in a bowl.

2. Serve the peanut butter in a separate bowl for dipping.

3. Enjoy!

Lunch

Turkey and Cheese Wrap with Carrot Sticks

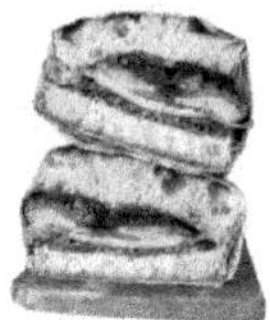

Ingredients

- 1 whole wheat wrap

- 2 oz sliced turkey breast

- 1 slice of cheddar cheese

- 1/4 cup shredded lettuce

- 1/4 cup sliced tomatoes

- Carrot sticks for serving

Preparation

1. Lay the whole wheat wrap on a flat surface.

2. Arrange the cheddar cheese, sliced tomatoes, shredded lettuce, and sliced turkey breast on top of the wrap.

3. Roll the wrap tightly, tucking in the ends.

4. Cut the wrap in half.

5. Serve with carrot sticks.

6. Enjoy!

Snack

Yogurt and Granola Parfait

Ingredients

- 1/2 cup plain Greek yogurt

- 1/4 cup granola

- 1/4 cup mixed berries (blueberries, raspberries, strawberries)

Preparation

1. In a small bowl or glass, layer the Greek yogurt, granola, and mixed berries.

2. Repeat the layers until all ingredients are used up.

3. Enjoy!

Dinner

Vegetable Stir-Fry with Tofu and Brown Rice

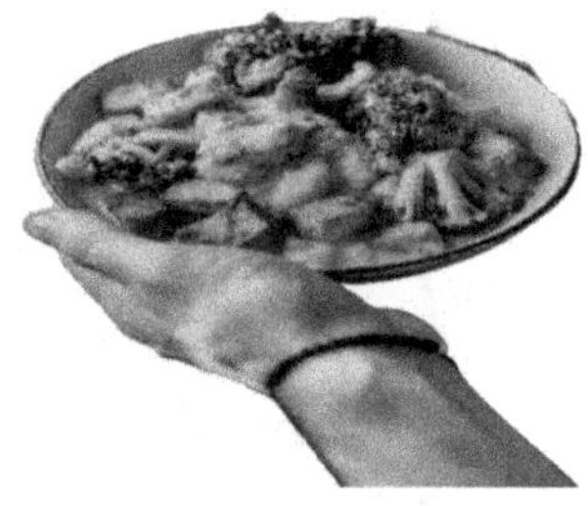

Ingredients

- 4 oz firm tofu, drained and cubed

- 1 cup mixed vegetables (bell peppers, onions, carrots, broccoli)

- 1/2 cup cooked brown rice

- 1 tbsp olive oil

- 1 tbsp soy sauce

Preparation

1. Set a nonstick skillet to medium-high heat.

2. Add the tofu cubes to the skillet and cook for 3 to 4 minutes, or until gently browned, stirring regularly.

3. Add the mixed veggies to the skillet and toss occasionally for 3 to 4 minutes, or until soft.

4. Drizzle the olive oil and soy sauce over the tofu and vegetables.

5. Cook for an additional 1-2 minutes, or until heated through.

6. Serve the stir-fry with the cooked brown rice.

7. Enjoy!

These meal plans and recipes can help individuals with high blood pressure improve their diet and control their blood pressure levels through healthy and delicious meals.

CHAPTER 16

Conclusion

The management of high blood pressure doesn't have to be challenging. By using natural treatments and changing a few simple but important aspects of your lifestyle, you may regain control over your health and well-being.

A successful diet should be well-balanced, full of fruits, vegetables, nutritious grains, and lean proteins, and free of processed foods and high sodium intake.

Routine exercise, such as brisk walking or swimming, increases overall vitality and strengthens your cardiovascular system. Additionally, implementing stress-reduction strategies like deep breathing exercises or meditation will help you on your way to having ideal blood pressure levels.

Keep in mind that managing your blood pressure is a long-term investment in your well-being. By accepting these natural therapies and implementing sustainable lifestyle adjustments, you are empowering yourself to live a bright, meaningful life free of the burdens of hypertension.

Begin your journey right away and discover the transformational power of these wise decisions, which will open the door to a healthier tomorrow.